Faehaa Azher Al-Mashhadane
Alyaa Azher Al-Mashhadane
Amer Abdul Rhman Taqa

Folic Acid Supplementation

Faehaa Azher Al-Mashhadane
Alyaa Azher Al-Mashhadane
Amer Abdul Rhman Taqa

Folic Acid Supplementation

A Review of the Known Advantages and Risks

Noor Publishing

Imprint
Any brand names and product names mentioned in this book are subject to trademark, brand or patent protection and are trademarks or registered trademarks of their respective holders. The use of brand names, product names, common names, trade names, product descriptions etc. even without a particular marking in this work is in no way to be construed to mean that such names may be regarded as unrestricted in respect of trademark and brand protection legislation and could thus be used by anyone.

Cover image: www.ingimage.com

Publisher:
Noor Publishing
is a trademark of
International Book Market Service Ltd., member of OmniScriptum Publishing Group
17 Meldrum Street, Beau Bassin 71504, Mauritius

Printed at: see last page
ISBN: 978-620-0-77619-8

Folic Acid Supplementation
A Review of the Known Advantages and Risks

By

Faehaa Azher Al-Mashhadane1, *,

Alyaa Azher Al-Mashhadane2,

Amer Abdul Rhman Taqa1, *

1Department of Dental Basic Sciences, University of Mosul, Mosul, Iraq

2Ministry of Health, Al-Salam Hospital, Mosul, Iraq

Abstract

Folate is required for metabolic processes and neural development.

The aim of this paper: To review the effects of folic acid supplementation before and throughout pregnancy on fetal development, summarize research needs with a focus on studying the effects of correct dosage folic acid.

Methods: Related publications were reviewed to determine and quantify associations of maternal use of folic acid before conception and during pregnancy as risk factor for Neural Tube Defects (NTD), Orofacial Clefts, ischemic heart diseases, Unmetabolised folic acid, Masking of B12 Deficiency Anemia and cancer. Evidence on maternal drug use before conception and during pregnancy as risk factor for developmental defect from epidemiological studies is still very limited. This review showed that a high prevalence of malformations and diseases that affect fetus could be related to the mother folic acid supplementation before and during pregnancy. Challenges in global prevalence estimation include quality of surveillance methods, geographic and socioeconomic factors, availability and use of folic acid, racial–ethnic and genetic factors, and limitations in education and access to care. For primary prevention of NTD in women with no prior affected pregnancy, 0.4 mg daily dose of folic acid was recommended and 4.0 mg daily dose was effective in preventing NTD in women with a prior affected pregnancy.

Also Maternal supplementation in early pregnancy reduces the risk of oral cleft in infants, evidence from the literature serve to reassure women planning a pregnancy to consume folic acid during the preconception period to protect against oral clefts. Several studies have confirmed that folic acid supplementation before Pregnancy was associated with a reduced risk of ischemic heart diseases; lower dietary folate intake during pregnancy was associated with increased risk. Folic acid may prevent or promote cancer development and progression depending on the timing of intervention.

In conclusion and based on the evidence evaluated, caution regarding under and/or over folic acid supplementation is warranted.

Keywords

Folic Acid, Pregnancy, Dose

Introduction

Available information suggests that currently over 47% of males and 59% of females use dietary supplements for health benefits, and the number of users is rapidly increasing.

However, numerous studies published over more than a decade have linked some supplements to no health benefits or even to adverse health effects. [1] Folic acid is a water-soluble B-complex vitamin. Reduced forms of folic acid are required for essential biochemical reactions that provide precursors for the synthesis of amino acids, purines, and DNA. [2]

Folate deficiency is relatively common, even though the deficiency is easily corrected by administration of folic acid.

Both animal and human studies have shown the essential role of folate during nervous system and brain development. [3].

Women are especially susceptible to folate deficiency during pregnancy, which is a period of rapid fetal growth, and high rates of cell division. Since the 1950s, folic acid supplementation has been known to prevent megaloblastic anemia during pregnancy.

In the 1990s, large randomized trials demonstrated that periconceptional folic acid supplementation can prevent neural tube defects (NTD) in the newborn infant. National health authorities in many countries recommend periconceptional folic acid supplementation, and some countries have introduced mandatory folate fortification of foods.

In Norway, folic acid supplementation of 400 µg/d is recommended from the time of planning a pregnancy to gestational week 12 as is a daily folate intake of 500 µg/d. This is in line with the Nordic Nutrition Recommendations[4].

Maternal folate status has also been associated with other adverse pregnancy outcomes such as preeclampsia, malformations such as orofacial clefts, spontaneous abortion, fetal death, fetal growth restriction and preterm delivery (PTD), although these results still remain inconclusive [5].

There may be an added benefit for adults, $N\,5-$ Methyltetrahydrofolate is required for the conversion of homocysteine to methionine. Impaired synthesis of $N\,5$ methyltetrahydrofolate results in elevated serum concentrations of homocysteine.

Data from several sources suggest a positive correlation between elevated serum homocysteine and occlusive vascular diseases such as ischemic heart disease and stroke. Clinical data suggest that the folate supplementation program has improved the folate status and reduced the prevalence of hyperhomocysteinemia in a population of middle-aged and older adults who did not use vitamin supplements [16].

In regards to risks of folic acid supplement, some opponents were concerned that increased folic acid intake in the general population would mask vitamin B 12 deficiency and increase the prevalence of neurologic disease in the elderly population. There is also concern based on observational and prospective clinical trials that high folic acid levels can increase the risk of some diseases, such as colorectal cancer, infant bronchiolitis and risk for autism spectrum disorder. [6-8].

In acknowledgment of this controversy, the FDA kept its requirements for folic acid supplementation at a somewhat low level.

Folic Acid and Neural Tube

Defects (NTD)

Neural tube defects (NTD), including spina bifida, anencephaly and encephalocele, result from incomplete neural tube closure during early embryogenesis. In addition to causing considerable perinatal mortality worldwide, NTD also give rise to infantile morbidity that often persists into adulthood.

Of all congenital malformations, NTD are among the most costly to treat, however they are unique in that more than two-thirds of cases are preventable by adequate intake of folic acid before and during the first trimester of pregnancy.

Neural tube defects (NTDs) are common and devastating congenital malformations of the central nervous system. The two most common, anencephaly (a total or partial absence of the brain tissue, skull, and overlying skin) and spina bifida (herniation of spinal cord, meninges, or both through a defect in the spine), comprise >90% of cases. Both arise from incomplete closure of the neural tube early in gestation, often before a woman is even aware that she might be pregnant. NTDs cause substantial morbidity and mortality for newborns and lead to staggering financial and emotional costs. Anencephaly results in inutero death, or death within a few days of birth.

In contrast, children afflicted with spina bifida suffer from physical disabilities including paralysis, bowel and bladder incontinence, learning disabilities, and excess mortality well into childhood and adult years, despite advances in medical and surgical care. There is strong evidence from clinical trials for a large preventive effect of folic acid on both recurrence and occurrence of NTDs. The strongest evidence for a preventive effect of high dose folic acid supplementation on recurrence of NTDs comes from the Medical Research Council (MRC) double-blinded randomized study, where women with a previous child with NTD were randomly assigned to groups of 4 mg folic acid, vitamins other than folic acid, vitamins with 4 mg folic acid, and placebo, taken daily at preconception and throughout the first trimester of pregnancy.

The study reported a significant reduction of about 72% in the rate of NTDs in the groups supplemented with folic acid compared to the other study groups.

No significant decreases in NTD recurrence were observed in the group receiving vitamins without folic acid, indicating that preventive effects were due the folic acid component. [9]

The World Health Organization recommends an RBC folate concentration greater than 400 ng/mL (906 nmol/L) in women of reproductive age to achieve the greatest reduction of NTDs. [10]

The NTD research provides a model for developing clinical trials aimed at assessing preventive effects of folic acid on recurrence and occurrence of oral clefts of direct relevance for clinical practice. A connection between NTDs and oral clefts can be supported by their similar time of occurrence during embryogenesis, their status as defects involving the midline of the embryo, their near identical population genetic characteristics (variable by geographic origin but with near identical recurrence risks and very similar birth prevalances overall), evidence of similar gene/environment contributions and the failure to identify any major genetic factor for either.

The mechanisms by which folic acid might prevent NTDs or other birth defects remain unexplained. It might be secondary to the need to overcome pharmaco genetic deficiencies in women who require higher baseline intakes to reach therapeutic levels. A recently proposed mechanism relates to antibodies to the folic acid receptor. The role of antibodies to the folate receptor has yet to be confirmed but could explain why some women respond to high doses of folic acid as this may be required to titer the effects of antibody bound to receptors. The pharmacologic rescue by high dose folic acid has been reported in a rat model where folate receptor antibodies induced intracellular folate deficiency associated with birth defects. [12]

Unfortunately, putting prevention into practice has been much more difficult than initially anticipated, and numerous controversies exist about some of the most important folic acid related issues facing women and public health authorities worldwide. Some of these contentious issues include the optimal dose of supplemental folic acid, the safety of folic acid, the optimal level of fortification (and if this is even effective), and the root causes of NTDs in different populations. The recommended daily allowance of folic acid for NTD prevention depends on obstetrical history.

For women with a prior history of NTD affected pregnancy, a 4.0 mg daily dose starting at least one month prior to conception and continuing throughout the first trimester is the current United States recommendation.

This dose was initially recommended in 1991 after the results of the MRC trial were published, which showed that a 4.0 mg daily dose was effective in preventing NTD in women with a prior affected pregnancy. For women with no prior affected pregnancy, the CDC broadened its guidelines in 1992 to include a recommended 0.4 mg daily dose for all women of childbearing age for primary prevention of NTD. This 0.4 mg dose was based on several case control and cohort studies as well as a 1992 Hungarian RCT that used 0.8 mg daily for primary prevention. In 1999, Berry *et al* provided additional evidence for 0.4 mg supplementation when a study carried out in China showed significant primary prevention of NTDs with that dose. Although it is possible that a lower dose could provide similar levels of protection as 4 mg, a randomized control trial assessing different doses will likely never be done due to ethical constraints. One fact making it difficult to measure effectiveness of folic acid fortification is that the proportion of NTDs that are actually folate sensitive is unknown. Decades of research have failed to show exactly how folic acid prevents NTDs.

Good sources of dietary folate that are often cited include legumes, orange juice, leafy green vegetables, broccoli, and whole grains. Unfortunately patient education materials often fail to distinguish between the wide variations in folate content in common foods. For example, broccoli has widely different folate values depending on whether it is cooked, raw, or frozen. [13]

In 1991, the Centers for Disease Control and Prevention recommended that women with a history of a prior NTDaffected pregnancy should consume 4000 µg of folic acid daily starting at the time they begin planning a pregnancy.

Subsequently, in 1992, the U.S. Public Health Service recommended that all women of childbearing age consume 400 µg of folic acid daily through fortification, supplementation, and diet to prevent NTDs. [14]

3. Folic Acid and Orofacial

Clefts (OFC)

Orofacial clefts (OFC) of the lip and palate are common birth defects of complex genetic and environmental etiology.

There is some suggestive evidence for a possible role of folic acid in prevention of OFC. However, several important questions remain unanswered including confirming whether folic acid prevents OFC, whether it prevents occurrence or recurrence or both, whether it prevents CL/P, CP or both, and identifying whether low or high doses are effective for prevention. Studies to date have provided mixed results particularly in regards to whether low or high dose folic acid can prevent primary occurrence. Most case-control observational studies indicating a preventive effect are likely to have evaluated low to moderate doses of (<1mg) folic acid though the majority did not measure or report the dose. One observational study found a decrease in CP with high dose folic acid, though no significant effect on CL/P. [9]

Insufficient intake of folic acid during the pregnancy has been suggested to increase the risk for CP Only. [15]

Orofacial clefts occur when the lips and/or the roof of the mouth do not fuse properly during development, leaving an opening; this occurs between 6 and 9 weeks of pregnancy.

Treatment involves plastic surgery, beginning approximately 3 months after birth and continuing into adolescence.

The effects on an individual's speech, hearing, appearance, and psychology can lead to long-lasting adverse outcomes for health and wellbeing. Even when repaired, complications such as persistent ear infections, speech impairments, facial deformities, and dental problems often remain.

A cleft lip and palate occurs in approximately one in 700 live births.

Cleft lip, with or without cleft palate, is most frequent in males and isolated cleft palate is most common in females.

Prevalence varies according to geography and ethnicity. The cause of cleft lip and palate is complex but involves both genetic and environmental factors. Genetic studies have demonstrated higher prevalence of cleft lip and palate in monozygotic twin pairs than in twins who are dizygotic, and in siblings in whom congenital anomalies exist.

Environmental factors have been implicated as contributors to cleft lip and palate 1 and include maternal exposure to: tobacco smoke; 3 alcohol; medicines such as anticonvulsant drugs, notably diazepam, phenytoin, and phenobarbital; 4 illicit drugs viral infection; and nutritional deficiencies. [1]

In humans, a finely choreographed cascade of gene expression, cell migration, cell transformation and apoptosis between 14 and 60 days post conception creates the soft and hard tissues of the face from the originating oropharyngeal membrane.

By 48 days the upper lip is continuous and by 60 days palatal shelf fusion completes facial embryogenesis.

Disruption of any of the tightly regulated processes occurring in this time frame by environmental and/or genetic abnormalities may then predispose to cleft lip and/or palate.[7]

Khan MFJ *et al* (2018) found that differences in DNA methylation, may impact lip fusion and warrant larger-scale replication. [11]

OFC include cleft lip with or without the palate (CL/P) as well as palate only (CP). CL/P and CP are sometimes differentiated in studies due to differences in embryologic origin and recurrence risks, but they are also combined in many studies due to common genetic and epidemiologic risks.

Recently the role for subphenotypes in clefts has also provided new insights into etiologies.

OFC occur in both isolated and non-isolated forms. Isolated or non-syndromic forms involve no other major structural or developmental impairments and represent the majority of cases with CL/P. The non-isolated or syndromic forms with CL/P occur due to more than 450 causes including chromosomal anomalies, single gene conditions, environmental exposures, and syndromes of unknown cause.

OFC impose significant health, psychosocial, and economic burdens, both at the individual and family levels, they are one of the most common birth defects with significant medical, psychosocial, and economic ramifications. [7]

There are suggestive results for decreased risks of cleft occurrence and recurrence with folic acid supplements taken at preconception and during pregnancy with a stronger evidence for higher than lower doses in preventing recurrence.

There is also well-documented effectiveness for folic acid in preventing neural tube defect occurrence at 0.4 mg and recurrence with 4 mg. Given the substantial burden of clefting on the individual and the family and the supportive data for the effectiveness of folic acid supplementation as well as its low cost, a randomized clinical trial of the effectiveness of high versus low dose folic acid for prevention of cleft recurrence is warranted. The complex etiology of cleft lip with or without cleft palate (oral clefts) affords ample opportunities to identify environmental and gene environment interactions and to establish programs for prevention. [12]

An effect of vitamin supplementation on the incidence of cleft lip and palate has been hypothesized for over 40years.

A number of subsequent studies reviewed by Czeizel and Munger have continued to suggest that folic acid and/or other micronutrients or vitamins, including vitamin A and vitamin B6, may be important in the etiology of clefts as well.

These studies strongly support further investigations of the role of vitamins and other environmental components in clefting and compel the determination as to whether interventional strategies can result in decreases. The results of these studies are suggestive of potential preventive effects of high dose folic acid on cleft recurrence.

The data from the Hungarian trials also support the notion of lack of preventive effects of low doses of folic acid on occurrence of oral clefts. The NTD model showing preventive effects of high and low dose folic acid on recurrence and occurrence respectively, and the suggestive results from interventional studies and observational studies for preventive effects of high doses on recurrence and occurrence of oral clefts strongly indicate that large doses of folic acid are needed. [13]

Exposure to folic acid antagonists such as antiepilepticdrugs and dihydrofolate reductase inhibitors was reported to double the odds for oral clefts. Animal studies also provide support for anti-teratogenic effects of prenatal folic acid supplementation and dietary folate. Peer et al. showed a 69% reduction in cortisone induced cleft palate occurrence in mice with folic acid injection; there was an 82% reduction with a combined treatment of folic acid and B6. Folic acid supplementation was also shown to decrease the frequency of retinoic acid induced cleft palate in mice by up to 92%, with suggested additive effects with methionine.

Procarbazine induced cleft palate was also reported to

decrease with folic acid supplementation in rats with potential dose and gender dependent effects of folic acid [12].

Only a handful of interventional studies have been conducted over the last 50 years to study the effect of folic acid supplementation on recurrence of oral clefts in mothers with a child with OFC. The decrease in OFC recurrence among the folic acid groups reported in these studies, independent of statistical significance, ranges from about 24 to 100%.

Conway (1958) reported no recurrent cleft cases among 59 births to mothers with history of OFC in previous births who received a multivitamin that included 0.5 mg of folic acid.

The recurrence rate in a group of 78 births to mothers who did not receive the supplement was 5.1%. Peer et al. (1964) reported a 53% reduction in the recurrence of OFC in a group of 176 women who received a multivitamin in addition to 5 mg folic acid and 10 mg vitamin B6 during the first pregnancy trimester, compared to a control group of 418 mothers.

In an extended study of Peer et al. (1964) with more supplemented women, Briggs (1976) reported a 35% reduction in recurrence of OFC, but a 65% reduction in CL/P recurrence.

Tolarova (1982) reported an 84% reduction in recurrence of CL/P in a group of 80 women who received a multivitamin and 10 mg of folic acid during three months before and after pregnancy (p=0.02), compared to a control group of 202 women. Using data on a larger sample that included women with CL/P (40% of intervened sample) and mothers of a child with CL/P, and the same intervention as Tolarova (1982), Tolarova and Harris (1995) reported a 66% reduction in recurrence of CL/P. Johnson and Little (2008) estimated a significant 67% reduction in CL/P recurrence based on these studies. These calculations are primarily descriptive given the array of interventions and populations used, but from an exploratory perspective, may be helpful for gauging expected treatment effects of folic acid to form hypotheses in clinical trials. The results of these studies are suggestive of potential preventive effects of high dose folic acid on cleft recurrence [9].

4. Folic Acid and Ischemic

Heart Diseases

Elevated plasma homocysteine (tHcy) has been associated with chronic disease of the vasculature including peripheral vascular, cerebrovascular and coronary heart disease, 1–3 as well as cognitive disease. New evidence also suggests an association of elevated plasma homocysteine with conditions affecting the vascular system in pregnancy, such as preeclampsia.

Several intervention studies have confirmed that folic acid will reduce homocysteine.

Large randomized clinical trials are now underway to determine whether folic acid supplements can diminish cardiovascular events by reducing plasma homocysteine. These prevention trials recruit patients with pre-existing cardiovascular disease [16].

The lowest dose of folic acid required to achieve effective reductions in homocysteine is controversial but important for food fortification policy given recent concerns about the potential adverse effects of overexposure to this vitamin.

Previous studies examined homocysteine-lowering in response to different folic acid doses but the results are inconsistent.

One of these studies investigated the effect of folic acid in the range 0.2–1 mg/d in IHD patients and showed that homocysteine decreased in a dose-dependent manner with increasing doses of folic acid up to a maximum effect (ie, 23% reduction) in response to 0.8 mg folic acid/d.

However, the study did not take into account initial homocysteine concentrations before randomization, which may have influenced the response [1].

Tighe p *et al.*, 2011 compared the effectiveness of 0.2 mg folic acid/d with that of 0.4 and 0.8 mg/d at lowering homocysteine concentrations over a 6-mo period.

They found that folic acid dose as low as 0.2 mg/d can, if administered for 6 mo, effectively lower homocysteine concentrations.

Higher doses may not be necessary because they result in no further significant lowering, whereas doses even lower than 0.2 mg/d may be effective in the longer term. Another dosefinding study, which stratified subjects on thebasis of pretreatment homocysteine, estimated that 0.4 mg folic acid/d was required to achieve 90% of the maximal homocysteine response.

Both of the aforementioned studies, together with 23 others, were then subjected to a meta-analysis that standardized for pretreatment homocysteine.

In conclusion, these results showed that a dose of folic acid as low as 0.2 mg/d can, if taken for 6 mo, effectively lower homocysteine concentrations. It was showed that higher doses of folic acid may not be necessary and, in support of the recent opinion expressed elsewhere, may be inappropriate given potential adverse effects of long-term exposure to high folic acid intakes. Previous trials may have overestimated the folic acid dose required because of too short an intervention period to observe a more complete response to lower doses [17].

5. Unmetabolised Folic Acid

Folic acid is a synthetic compound that when ingested is converted by dihydrofolate reductase to the dihydrofolate and then to the tetrahydrofolate form of folate; these reduced compounds are identical to those that would arise from ingestion of natural folate. However, large oral doses of folic acid can overwhelm this mechanism, and conversion of folic acid to reduced folate is bypassed, which leads to a build-up of folic acid in the serum. Unmetabolized serum folic acid (UMFA) does not arise after consumption of naturally occurring folate.

Very little is known about the metabolism and biological effects of UMFA. Some have hypothesized that the presence of UMFA may be a contributing factor in safety concerns associated with high intakes of folic acid. [18]

Research to date suggests that the enzymatic reduction and methylation of folic acid during its absorption in the intestine or its first pass through the liver is dose-dependent.

Hence oral folic acid above certain threshold doses saturates the normal intestinal absorptive mechanisms and results in unmetabolised folic acid in serum as well as the normal metabolite 5-methyltetrahydrofolate. This has been demonstrated at oral doses in the region of 200 µg and 266 µg. In a more recent paper it was shown that repeated consumption of physiological amounts of folic acid lead to the accumulation of unmetabolised folic acid in serum. It has also been demonstrated that passive consumption of folic acid in foodstuffs by pregnant women leads to the appearance of unmetabolised folic acid in foetal cord blood.

While these studies examined the acute serum response to folic acid, none have investigated the effect after a prolonged period of exposure to the vitamin. [19]

Folic acid has the potential to mask the early haematological manifestations of pernicious anemia. This has been demonstrated experimentally and clinically. Other safety considerations of excess folic acid consumption highlighted by the FDA include potential unknown risks for pregnant women, and persons on antiepileptic and anti-folate medication. The FDA also noted the uncertainties regarding the effects of chronic exposure in children, whose requirements for folate are lower than those of adults. Furthermore evidenced based and hypothetical concerns include the potential to promote cancer and the recent hypothesis that exposure of the fetus to excess folic acid may favor the selection of the Methylentetrahydrofolate polymorphism, associated with a range of debilitating illnesses.

To date no studies have examined the effect of long-term consumption of folic acid on unmetabolised folic acid in serum.

The accumulation of folic acid after consumption of fortified bread repeatedly over only one 8-hour period provides justification for this.

Folic acid normally is reduced to tetrahydrofolate following uptake by the liver. If the body's ability to reduce folic acid is exceeded, unmetabolized folic acid will be found circulating in the blood.

One experimental study suggested that unmetabolized folic acid would be found after consuming a bolus of >200 µg of folic acid.

Intakes exceeding this threshold would be common through the use of supplements or fortified foods such as breakfast cereals, but unlikely would be reached through intake of folic acid from mandatory U.S. fortification levels alone. Because folic acid has been a long-standing component of over-the-counter supplements and prenatal vitamins, if looked for, unmetabolized folic acid would have been found among a large proportion of the U.S. population for decades.

Only recently has the laboratory equipment needed to measure circulating unmetabolized folic acid become available.

Unmetabolized folic acid has been found among many groups examined—from older U.S. adults to the cord blood from newly delivered infants. It has been hypothesized that unmetabolized folic acid is related to cognitive impairment among seniors, although the findings might have been confounded by patients with pernicious anemia.

Currently, there are no definitive studies that have found health effects from exposure to unmetabolized folic acid. [20]

6. Masking of B12 Deficiency

Anemia

Historically, concerns surrounding folic acid use have focused on the possibility that folic acid could mask the anemia caused by vitamin B12 deficiency.

Early case reports (1940–1960) suggested ≥5000 µg of folic acid daily could mask a vitamin B12 deficiency by preventing the development of anemia.

In turn, this could delay the diagnosis of an underlying vitamin B12 deficiency and thereby allow vitamin B12 deficiency-associated neuropathies to progress.

It is recognized that the diagnosis of a vitamin B12 deficiency and/or response to treatment should be dependent on a series of vitamin B12 blood status indicators and not solely on hematological indices which may not be reliable.

The IOM concluded in 1998 that there was no clear evidence of folate-induced neurotoxicity in humans. Several studies both before and after fortification have examined this issue and concluded that, at current recommended intakes, there is little evidence of masking or exacerbation of neuropathies.[17]

Additionally, the 2007 guidelines from the Motherisk program and the Society of Obstetricians and Gynecologists of Canada call for 5mg/d for women with a variety of medical and social indications, including minority status, epilepsy, obesity, substance abuse, poor medication compliance, and lack of birth control.

These recommendations are not reflective of those that are generally available in other jurisdictions, however. This 5 mg/d recommendation is notable because it is so far above most other recommendations and because it well exceeds the generally accepted tolerable upper limit (TUL) of folic acid of 1.0 mg daily. This limit is based on concerns of possible masking of B12 deficiency anemia (pernicious anemia) through the use of high dose folic acid, leading to the progression of irreversible neurologic defects resulting from B12 deficiency. Studies performed in the 1950s showed the level of folic acid needed to correct the B12 deficiencyrelated anemia was about 5.0 g per   day. The Institute of Medicine then established the TUL at a somewhat arbitrary level 5 times lower than this, at 1 mg per   day. Of note, vitamin B12 levels are now routinely and easily measured in patients with unexplained neurological symptoms.

Additionally, studies performed post-fortification have shown no significant change in B12 levels after fortification, nor has fortification increased the percentage of people with B12 deficiency presenting in the absence of anemia. These observations are important for two reasons. The first is that a "safety concern" is frequently mentioned throughout the literature as an argument against widespread folic acid use.

Indeed, potential masking of B12 deficiency was a key reason United Kingdom health regulators decided against fortification there in 2002; thishas likewise been a contentious issue in Australia, Switzerland, and other countries that continue to debate fortification.

Secondly, the TUL was a main factor behind the fortification policy implemented in the United States. The fortification level was chosen to ensure that while the majority of people would get an extra 0.1 g/d, almost no one would cross the 1.0 mg/d threshold.[13]

7. Folic Acid and Cancer

Folate may prevent or promote cancer development and progression depending on the timing of intervention. Intrauterine exposure to folic acid has drastically increased in North America due to mandatory fortification and supplemental use of folic acid, which may influence the risk of breast cancer in the offspring. [21]

There is growing evidence that one adverse effect of folic acid fortification programs is an increased risk of colorectal cancer within populations. The complexity of folate dependent, one-carbon metabolism and the heterogeneity that exists between individuals with respect to the enzymes involved in the anabolic pathways, are explored. [7]

Folic acid may facilitate the preliminary stages of specific malignant processes.

Hospitalization rates for colon cancer among men and women age 45 and older in Chile more than doubled after folic acid fortification was introduced in the country. Additionally, two Norwegian studies, the Norwegian Vitamin Trial and the Western Norway B Vitamin. Intervention Trial, found that supplementation with

800mcg/d of folic acid, B12, and B6 for more than three years increased the risk of lung cancer by 21%.

An analysis of these latter two studies, designed to study the effects of higher dose folic acid and vitamin B12 on reducing cardiovascular deaths by lowering plasma homocysteine levels, showed that high dose (synthetic) folic acid supplementation unexpectedly may increase cancer and all-cause mortality.

It is important to note, however, that the dose used in these two trials is twice that recommended on an international basis for pregnancy-related intakes. Systematic studies of the safety of high doses of folic acid are lacking, and it is axiomatic that absence of data does not imply assurance of safety.

No single 2 agency is tasked with the responsibility of monitoring the long-term or overall safety of the fortification program. The lack of systematic safety studies means uncertainty about which outcomes are the most sensitive predictors of risk. The issue is proving to be of great urgency to researchers, governments, and industry, given the level of mandatory folic acid fortification in the United States and other countries and the many years of education on the health benefits associated with folic acid that has been directed at consumers. [13]

Several reports suggest that folate has a procarcinogenic effect.

Folate has a unique role because its coenzymes are needed for *de novo* purine and thymine nucleotide biosynthesis. Antifolates, such as methotrexate, are used in cancer treatment. Using a meta-analysis weighted for the duration of folic acid (pteroylglutamic acid) supplementation.

The cancer incidence of six previously published large prospective folic acid-supplementation trials in men and women were analyzed.

These articles were carefully selected from over 1100 identified using PubMed search.

These analyses suggest that cancer incidences were higher in the folic acid-supplemented groups than the non-folic acidsupplemented groups (relative risk = 1.21 [95% confidence interval: 1.05–1.39]).

Folic acid supplementation trials should be performed with careful monitoring of cancer incidence.

Solid monitoring systems to detect side effects, including increase in cancer risk, should be established before the initiation of folic acid supplementation trials. [22]

Evidence has emerged identifying folic acid supplementation

as a potential risk factor for cancer development or progression. Long-term folic acid supplementation has been shown to increase the risk of prostate cancer development by three-fold. Sarcosine is a byproduct of folate metabolism and has been proposed as a biomarker for aggressive prostate cancer phenotypes.

The effects of physiologically relevant levels of folic acid on *in vitro* prostate cancer cell growth and invasion had been studied, it was demonstrated that higher levels of folic acid can have the effect of increasing both of these biological processes,folic acid and prostste cancer.

Previous epidemiological studies of circulating folate concentration and colorectal cancer have reported inconsistent results.

Takata; *et al* (2014) evaluated associations of pre-diagnostic plasma folate concentration with colorectal cancer risk in a case-control study nested within the Shanghai Men's Health Study (2002-2010).

They found that plasma folate concentration was positively associated with colorectal cancer risk. [23].

Kawakita D *et al* evaluated the association between folate intake and HNC risk using prospective cohort data from the Prostate, Lung, Colorectal, and Ovarian (PLCO) cancer screening trial.

Their findings provide evidence of the protective role of dietary folate intake on head and neck cancer risk. [24]

There is strong evidence that low folate status promotes cancer, especially colorectal cancer.As noted in the NTP report, there is both preclinical data from rodent models and human observational and clinical evidence to indicate that inadequate folate intake from all sources is associated with increased cancer risk.

Because folate cofactors are required for nucleotide biosynthesis and for generating activated methyl groups that modify chromatin and affect gene expression, low-folate status has been demonstrated to decrease rates of nucleotide biosynthesis and impair chromatin methylation.

Hence, low-folate status promotes genome instability and DNA mutation rates and alters the methylation patterns in the genome that affect the expression of tumor suppressor genes. There is strong consensus in the scientific community that folate deficiency increases risk for certain cancers.

Elevated folate status has been proposed to promote tumorigenesis from preexisting foci of neoplasia and accelerate the growth of established tumors.

The biological premise underlying this hypothesis relates to the role of folate in the synthesis of nucleotides for DNA synthesis in rapidly dividing cells and the use of antifolate chemotherapeutics (methotrexate, pemetrexed, and 5-flurouracil, among others) that target and inhibit folate-dependent enzymes and inhibit cell proliferation. Antifolates have been used successfully in the treatment of many types of cancer, and some postulate that, by increasing nucleotide synthesis for cellular proliferation, folate from all sources could accelerate tumor growth.

However, evidence demonstrating a dose–response relationship between folate status and/or folate/folic acid intake within the normal human exposure ranges and increased rates of tumor growth *in vivo* are lacking, and it has not been established whether folate availability is rate limiting in tumor growth in individuals with adequate folate status [25].

8. The tolerable upper intake level for folic acid

There is no UL for natural reduced folates found in foods. The UL for the pro-vitamin folic acid was established to avoid a delayed diagnosis of vitamin B_{12} deficiency, as assessed by hematological indices, and thereby minimize the risk of neurological complications in vitamin B_{12}-deficient individuals. The IOM stated, "The weight of the limited but suggestive evidence that excessive folate intake may precipitate or exacerbate neuropathy in vitamin B_{12}-deficient individuals justifies the selection of this end point as the critical end point for the development of a UL for foliate.

The IOM was careful to note that there was not sufficient evidence to establish a UL on the basis of a no-observed-adverse-effect level (NOAEL) but rather on the basis of a lowest-observed-adverse-effect level (LOAEL).

The LOAEL was set at 5 mg/day on the basis of several case reports and small observational studies showing that, at doses of 5 mg/day folic acid and above, there were more than 100 reported cases (from more than 20 studies) of neurological progression in patients with pernicious anemia, compared with fewer than eight cases in studies administering less than 5 mg/day oral folic acid.

As stated by the IOM, "The LOAEL of 5 mg/day of folate was divided by an uncertainty factor of 5 to obtain the UL for adults of 1 mg/day or 1000 µg/day of folate from supplements or fortified food. A UL of 1000 µg/day is set for all adults rather than just for the elderly because of (1) the devastating and irreversible nature of the neurological consequences of a delayed diagnosis and treatment of a vitamin B_{12} deficiency, (2) data suggesting that pernicious anemia may develop at a younger age in some racial or ethnic groups, and (3) uncertainty about the occurrence of vitamin B_{12} deficiency in younger age groups."

According to the IOM, "the prevalence of vitamin B_{12} deficiency in females in the childbearing years is very low and the consumption of supplemental folate at or above the UL in this subgroup is unlikely to produce adverse effects, although exceptions might include vegetarians, subsets of the population that have low dietary meat intake, and chronic users of proton pump inhibitors.

Hematological indices are not commonly used to assess vitamin B_{12} deficiency, as they have been replaced with the use of serum biomarkers; hence, the basis for the UL

for folic acid, which is based on hematological
assessment of vitamin B_{12} deficiency, is less meaningful
today relative to when it was established nearly 20 years
ago. [25]

9. Conclusion

Maternal folic acid supplementation prior to and during pregnancy should be kept as low as possible, higher doses of may not be necessary.

The current use of folic acid supplement during pregnancy potentially exposes pregnant women and their unborn children to too much folic acid.

Neural tube defects (NTD) are major congenital malformations affecting births worldwide. Regardless of the etiology of different neural tube defects, correct-dose folic acid prophylaxis must be recommended in all cases. Folic acid holds great potential as a critical and convenient therapeutic intervention for neural engineering and regenerative medicine.

Consequently, Efforts will assist in both global prevention of NTD and periodic evaluation of folic acid interventions for NTD reduction.

Further observations are required to establish the role of folic acid in fetal epigenetic modifications and to demonstrate the physiological doses of folic acid that can be recommended for primary prevention trials of conditions postulated to be folic acid-related.

Overall, the totality of the evidence of the literature fully
supports the benefits of mandatory folic acid fortification
in NTD prevention.

Furthermore, there are no established risks for adverse
consequences resulting from existing mandatory folic
acid fortification programs that have been implemented in
many countries.

Current folic acid fortification programs have been shown
to support public health in populations, and the exposure
levels are informed by and adherent to the precautionary
principle. Additional research is needed to assess the
health effects of folic acid supplement use when the
current UL for folic acid is exceeded.

References

[1] Soni MG, Thurmond TS, Miller ER, Spriggs T, Bendich, A and Omaye ST. Safety of Vitamins and Minerals: Controversies and Perspective. TOXICOLOGICAL SCIENCES 2010; 118 (2): 348–355.

[2] Zhao M, Chen Y. H, Chen X, Dong X. T. Folic acid supplementation during pregnancy protects against lipopolysaccharide-induced neural tube defects in mice. Toxicology Letters 2014; 224 (2): 201-208.

[3] Schmidt RJ, Tancredi DJ, Ozonoff S, Hansen RL, Hartiala J,
Allayee H, Schmidt LC, Tassone F, and Hertz-Picciotto I. Maternal periconceptional folic acid intake and risk of autism spectrum disorders and developmental delay in the CHARGE (CHildhood Autism Risks from Genetics and Environment) case-control study. Am J Clin Nutr 2012; 96: 80–9.

[4] Li Z, Ye R, Zhang L, Li H, Liu J, Ren A. Periconceptional folic acid supplementation and the risk of preterm births in China: a large prospective cohort study. Int J Epidemiol 2014.

[5] Sengpiel V, Bacelis J, Myhre R, Myking S, Devold Pay A, Haugen M. Folic acid supplementation, dietary

folate intake during pregnancy and risk for spontaneous preterm delivery: a prospective observational cohort study. BMC Pregnancy and Childbirth 2013; 13: 160.

[6] Veeranki SP, Gebretsadik T, Dorris SL, Mitchel EF, Hartert TV, Cooper WO, Tylavsky FA, Dupont W, Hartman TJ,Carroll KN. Association of folic Acid supplementation during pregnancy and infant bronchiolitis. Am J Epidemiol 2014; 15; 179 (8): 938-46.

[7] Jennings BA, Willis G. How folate metabolism affects colorectal cancer development and treatment; a story of heterogeneity and pleiotropy. Cancer Lett. 2014 Mar 12: S0304-3835 (14) 00131-1.

[8] Wiens D, DeSoto MC. Is High Folic Acid Intake a Risk Factor for Autism?-A Review. Brain Sci. 2017 10; 7 (11).

[9] Wehby G, Jeffrey C. Murray. Folic Acid and Orofacial Clefts:A Review of the Evidence. Oral Dis. 2010; 16 (1): 11–19.

[10] Viswanathan M, Treiman KA, Doto JK *et al*. Folic Acid Supplementation: An Evidence Review for the U.S. Preventive Services Task Force. AHRQ Publication 2017 No.14-05214-EF-1.

[11] dKhan MFJ, Little J, Mossey PA, Steegers-Theunissen RP,Autelitano L, Lombardo I, Andreasi RB, Rubini M.

Evaluating LINE-1 methylation in cleft lip tissues and its association with early pregnancy exposures. Epigenomics 2018 Jan; 10 (1): 105-113.

[12] Wehby G, Goco N, Moretti-Ferreira D, Felix T, Richieri-CostaA, Padovani C, Queiros F, Guimaraes CV, Pereira R, LitaveczS, Hartwell T, Chakraborty H, Javois L and Murray JC. Oralcleft prevention program (OCPP). BMC Pediatrics 2012; 12:184.

[13] Dunlap B, Shelke K, Salem SA, Keith LG. Folic acid and human reproduction—ten important issues for clinicians. J Exp Clin Assist Reprod 2011; 8: 2.

[14] Crider KS, Bailey LB and Berry RJ. Folic Acid Food Fortification—Its History, Effect, Concerns, and Future Directions. Nutrients 2011; *3*: 370-384.

[15] Tettamanti L, Avantaggiato A, Nardone M, Silvestre-Rangil J,Tagliabue A. Cleft palate only: current concepts. Oral Implantol (Rome) 2017; 10 (1): 45-52.

[16] Daly S, Mills JL, Molloy AM, Conly M, Mcpartlin J, Lee YJ,Young PB, Kirke PN, Weir DJ and Scott JM. Low-dose folic acid lowers plasma homocysteine levels in women of childbearing age. QJ Med 2002; 95: 733–740.

[17] Tighe P, Ward M, McNulty H, Finnegan O, Dunne A, Strain JJ, Molloy AM, Duffy M, Pentieva K, and Scott JM. A dosefinding trial of the effect of long-term folic

acid intervention: implications for food fortification policy. Am J Clin Nutr 2011; 93: 11–8.

[18] Bailey RL, Mills JL, Yetley EA, Gahche JJ, Pfeiffer CM, Dwyer JT, Dodd KW, Sempos CT, Betz JM, and Picciano MF. Unmetabolized serum folic acid and its relation to folic acid intake from diet and supplements in a nationally representative sample of adults aged 60 y in the United States.Am J Clin Nutr 2010; 92: 383–9.

[19] Sweeney MR, McPartlin J and Scott J. Folic acid fortificationand public health: Report on threshold doses above which unmetabolised folic acid appear in serum. BMC Public Health2007; 7: 41.

[20] Crider KS, Bailey LB and Berry RJ. Folic Acid Food Fortification—Its History, Effect, Concerns, and Future Directions. Nutrients 2011; 3: 370-384.

[21] Sie KY, Chen J, Sohn KJ, Croxford R, Thompson LU, Kim Y. Folic acid supplementation provided in utero and during lactation reduces the number of terminal end buds of the developing mammary glands in the offspring. Cancer letters 2009; 280 (1): 72-77.

[22] Baggott JE, Oster RA, Tamura T. Meta-analysis of cancer risk in folic acid supplementation trials. Cancer Epidemiology 2012; 36 (1): 78–81.

[23] Takata Y, Shrubsole MJ, Li H, Cai Q, Gao J, Wagner C, Wu J,Zheng W, Xiang YB, Shu XO. Plasma

folate concentrationsand colorectal cancer risk: a case-control study nested withinthe Shanghai Men's Health Study. Int J Cancer 2014.

[24] Kawakita D, Lee YA, Gren LH, Buys SS, La Vecchia C, Hashibe M. The impact of folate intake on the risk of head and neck cancer in the prostate, lung, colorectal, and ovarian cancer screening trial (PLCO) cohort. Br J Cancer 2017.

[25] Field MS and Stover PJ. Safety of folic acid. Ann N Y Acad Sci. 2018 ; 1414(1): 59–71.

Table of Contents

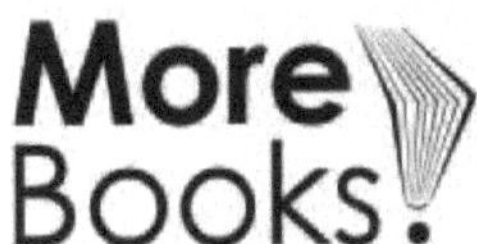

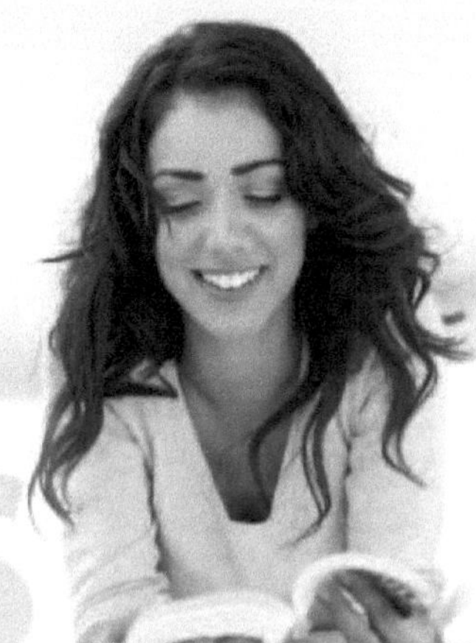

I **want** morebooks!

Buy your books fast and straightforward online - at one of world's fastest growing online book stores! Environmentally sound due to Print-on-Demand technologies.

Buy your books online at
www.morebooks.shop

Kaufen Sie Ihre Bücher schnell und unkompliziert online – auf einer der am schnellsten wachsenden Buchhandelsplattformen weltweit! Dank Print-On-Demand umwelt- und ressourcenschonend produziert.

Bücher schneller online kaufen
www.morebooks.shop

KS OmniScriptum Publishing
Brivibas gatve 197
LV-1039 Riga, Latvia
Telefax: +371 686 204 55

info@omniscriptum.com
www.omniscriptum.com

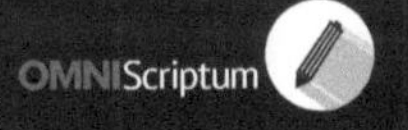

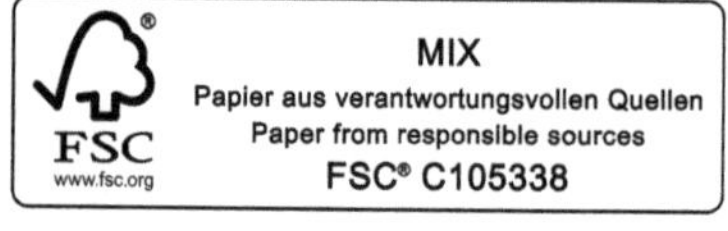

FSC
www.fsc.org
MIX
Papier aus verantwortungsvollen Quellen
Paper from responsible sources
FSC® C105338